FIT, FAT AND HAPPY

By Roz Baker

This book is dedicated to:

Everyone who is working on being their best self

Everyone who ever exercised with me in class

Family and friends who support, inspire and motivate me

My husband, Halis, for always being there.

Thank you!

INTRODUCTION

You are going to buy this book, or maybe, you're just thinking about it. Who needs another book on health and exercise? I hear you. I got sick of the fad diets and the "you can do it too" mantras being touted from folks who "did it" themselves.

Let's face it. If you want to be fat and you don't care about your health, MORE POWER TO YOU! Eat all the fat, sugar and junk you want. Don't exercise and die early. If you're lucky, you'll die fast.

Now if your mouth dropped open and you're saying to yourself, "I do not WANT to be fat. I am not lazy. I do care, but THIS WEIGHT THING IS VERY HARD".

YOU ARE SO RIGHT!

To all of those people who say to you (because they say it to me) "just stop eating", yeah right. That's like saying, "just say no" to a drug addict. People who don't enjoy eating the way I do cannot understand the high I get from devouring my favorite foods. And I have cut back, I swear. But the truth is, I enjoy good food. I like to eat bread. No butter—just plain bread, especially that sweet Hawaiian style used to make French toast. Every now and then I want a big, juicy cheeseburger with grilled onions and French fries. A close friend of mine just couldn't understand why I was so big because I work out all the time. When I told her "I like to eat", she said, "Then just eat vegetables". EXCUSE ME. Unless the veggie is batter-dipped and fried, I ain't interested.

So… What's a fat person to do? First,

STOP TRIPPING!

Second, please buy this book. Read it. I promise you there are no gimmicks and everything is true and backed by real, universally accepted science. (I did throw in a few personal theories, but they are clearly marked.) There is useful information you may not have known already and maybe just one fact that might make loving yourself—as you are, easier. And hopefully it will make you laugh.

Oh yeah, who is this Roz Baker? Well I'm an aerobics instructor/personal trainer certified by ACE (American Council on Exercise) who has lived most of my life on the plump side, been active all my life and is hoping that by sharing my experiences and knowledge I just might help someone else be *Fit Fat & Happy.*

CHAPTER ONE

WHAT IS FAT ANYWAY?

In the Random House College Dictionary (the old one which is actually printed), the definition of fat is *1. having too much adipose tissue; 2. plump, well fed.* Reading down, more definitions are *7. profitable as an office or position 9. wealthy, prosperous, rich 18. the richest or best part of anything.*

When did fat become a bad thing? A man I once dated, said, "angels are built like you", (referring to the winged childlike cherubs depicted in some religious paintings) "and that's a good thing". Okay, it was probably a line to get in my panties, but it made me feel good. Once upon a time, being fat signified you had so much money you never went hungry. Fat was preferred to skinny. A bigger woman looked strong and able. Now the only fat that's good is spelled "phat" ... Translation: Pretty Hot And Tempting.

Whatever the case, the truth is our bodies are programmed to like high-calorie foods. Back-in-the-day, one might have needed extra adipose tissue to get through a period of no food.

Americans around today had ancestors who survived slow hunting seasons or ruined crops with efficient metabolisms. And if you still have a very efficient metabolism (I think that sounds so much better than slow) keeping weight low isn't easy.

There are several reasons why some people can eat everything and stay at a "normal" weight while people like me can smell a donut and gain weight. Some studies have shown some people have a genetic dysfunction, which causes their body to not realize when it's full. Other studies say that's not true. Some bodies could be more efficient at storing fat, so that's what they do. Whether it is because of an increase in insulin production with insensitivity, (insulin is there, but the body can't use it efficiently) or a high level of the enzyme lipoprotein lipase, who knows? Who cares? The bottom line is, it's like that and that's the way it is.

After carefully reviewing my eating behavior and exercise I came to this conclusion. I eat too much to be skinny or even slim. I exercise regularly and although I don't eat a lot, I ingest too many calories to get slim. My genetics, my emotions,

Mercury rising in Jupiter... whatever... For me, it's like that and that's the way it is. I am a typical American and most Americans eat too many calories *although they don't eat a lot of food.* On top of that, most Americans don't exercise at all and when they do, not effectively. The result is almost half of the population in the United States is considered overweight or fat.

Unfortunately, fat people are viewed as the ugly stepchildren of society. Everybody wants to fix them; feel sorry for them and help them become thin and happy. After all, everybody who is overweight wants to be thin and happy.

REALLY!

There are hordes of commercials enticing you to eat a cheesy pizza while the next advertising campaign tells you nothing tastes as good as thin feels. It's enough to make you crazy.

Personally, I am sick of it. I have a theory. The nature of capitalism is to keep everybody buying. (I'm not mad at 'em.) To keep folks buying, there must be wants. To keep folks wanting, you sell them something almost unattainable or something they will always need. Toilet paper falls into the "always need" category. Some companies would have you believe you "need" to look like a body builder or an ultra thin model to have a perfect life. A little on the "almost unattainable" side.

We fat people are not stupid. Most of us think, I will never look like that, so why bother trying? Well, this is where I hope to change your attitude. Exercise will help you, even if you NEVER lose weight. Shaping up doesn't mean get someone else's shape. It means shaping your shape. Work with what you have and with what you like to do.

Back to fat. Why do we have it? It's necessary. It cushions your organs and insulates the body. Fat is our energy storage. The fit average man could have 7 – 20% body fat; women 12 – 25% (we have babies so we need more). Healthy fat percentages can go up to 30% for women. You can be tested to find out your percentages and if you need a number for comparisons sake, more power to you. I find it easier to look in the mirror and tell if I'm over-fat. If you have more energy storage, it simply means you take in more calories than you burn off on a regular basis. So what? Well…

Let me state the obvious:

BEING OVERWEIGHT IS UNHEALTHY.

Our heart and lungs supply oxygen and nutrients via the blood stream to every cell. When they have to carry supplies for an extra load, they tend not to last as long. Being over fat may cause some types of cancer. Extra weight is also hard on the skeletal system. So, what's a fat person to do?

Exercise to make your body as strong as possible, so it can work as well as it can, for as long as it can.

SAY WHAT?

Exercise to make your body as strong as possible, so it can work as well as it can for as long as it can. You thought this was an anti-exercise book?

CHAPTER 2

Why do I Have to Exercise?

The short answer is "because it's good for you!" Go ahead and smack the image you have of a skinny, bouncy-looking, twenty-something-year-old aerobic teacher smiling at you as she says "you can do it". Let's get back to basics.

Your body, besides carrying your spirit, is a chemical and physical exchange of energy. We take in energy, (in the form of calories), several different processes go on to regenerate your cells and then we excrete the waste product. All super-scientific-minded peeps might want to go into the atoms, with the nucleus and the circling protons, electrons and neutrons, and the fact that when two atoms get together, they match up protons and electrons and kick out what they don't need... If this doesn't sound vaguely familiar from high school chemistry, don't worry about it. It's really not important to the end product. Let's just simplify things by saying your metabolism is the collective term for all of these energy exchanges happening in your body.

Here's an easier way to visualize this concept:

Remember the sperm and the egg? They meet, form a cell, it splits and so on and so on and... Well soon into this process, some cells become bone cells, some muscle cells and once you stop growing, the cells just replace themselves.

Exfoliating the skin. Women, (and some men). know that to keep skin looking healthy, you have to scrub off the dead skin cells. There are dead skin cells because skin is constantly regenerating itself. Aging slows the process down and some cells get damaged along the way (as in a scar), but it still works.

Hair is the by-product of a working metabolism. So are fingernails. That is why when we cut them, they regrow. The body constantly regenerates by replenishing old muscle cells, bone cells and blood cells. Get a scratch? In weeks, all traces of it are gone due regenerating skin cells. This is our beautiful bodies at work.

Exercise stimulates the metabolism, which is a very important thing for a healthy body...regardless of its size. The body does its job better, (and its job is regenerating cells),

when you exercise, *even if you don't lose weight!*

Your body is like a car in some ways. If you take a car, put it in the garage for a year and come back to it, it won't start. The gaskets, which usually have oil splashing on them to keep them lubricated, dry out. The car is going to need servicing before it will run and it may never run the same, but it will still work.

Exercise is a measured, goal-oriented way to safely and correctly stimulate the metabolism and keep it in good working order. There are three areas of exercise needed by the body: Muscular, cardiovascular and flexibility.

Muscle exercise helps develop and maintain muscle strength. We all need muscle strength, even if the hardest thing we do is lift groceries into the car.

Cardiovascular exercise is make-sure-your-oxygen-transport-system-is-in-peak-condition exercise. It is extremely important in keeping your heart, lungs and blood vessels working efficiently.

Third and equally important is flexibility exercise. Every movement your body makes is the result of a muscle contracting or extending, usually around a joint. These joints like to be moved through their full range of motion on a regular basis. It keeps them "oiled" and less prone to injury. Let's look at that car again. You open the door partially all the time because the parking spots are always too damn close. One day you're in a parking lot and, a miracle of miracles, you can open the door all the way and not dent the car next to you. You go for it… grab that handle and pull it just past the point where you usually stop and eek! You hear this awful, make-your-skin-crawl screech. That's what your body joints do when they aren't open and closed all the way on a regular basis. Of course, they don't screech (well, they might). They do however, get stiff and unfortunately are more prone to injury. Stretching exercises help keep the muscles, tendons and joints of your body healthy.

Those are the three types of exercises needed to keep the body healthy and running efficiently, regardless of its size. So even if you're carrying around a little extra stored energy (or a lot of stored energy) your body will work better if you do all three types of exercises regularly. If you are beanpole skinny, you still need exercise to keep your body healthy.

Well, have I convinced you? Oh yes, it is worth it…What? It doesn't take that much time… Having a job where you walk a lot is not the same… You don't *have* to go to a gym…

CHAPTER THREE

Excuses, Excuses

It amazes me how many people decide, for whatever reason, not to exercise. I don't understand it. No one complains about brushing their teeth, it's just something you have to do to keep them. So why not treat your body the same way? You need to exercise to keep the body healthy. Period.

As an instructor, over the years I've heard over a dozen excuses. I'll list some of my favorite.

I HATE EXERCISING!

Why? Your body needs it. It actually craves it. When you are sitting around the house feeling like you want to "do something" your body is telling you it needs to expel some of this energy it's storing.

Perhaps you have a bad memory about exercise. Seriously. You'd be surprised at how something like being the last one picked for the softball team in eighth grade sticks with you; or being the last one picked for the volleyball team. I was the last one to get picked for teams in elementary and high school

and at the neighborhood park. And yes, it hurt my feelings. But

I got over it.

Perhaps you associate exercise with some sort of ritual

someone else imposed on you. In high school, I used to hate

these grotesque blue uniforms we had to wear. And on top of

that, they had to be cleaned and pressed. Who irons something

to sweat in? Why clean shoes that are going to get scuffed up

anyway? Many of my friends hated gym for that very reason

and consequently hated exercise. They would get a failing

grade in PE (Physical Education) because they didn't want to

be bothered. Then their GPA would be negatively affected and

so this "hate" of exercise begins. Years later, I understand. But

associating the "ritual" with the deed is not fair. You are not

being graded, you don't have to dress a certain way and you

NEED exercise. Get over it. Find your people and work out with

them. They are out here. Wear what you want as long as it

provides some support where needed. Even if it's wrinkled and

has a little stain, nobody cares. Don't be smelly though—if you

are indoors with other people—just common courtesy.

If hating exercise is your excuse, I urge you to examine your history and see just what makes you hate exercise. You probably just hate someone or something in your past you unjustly connect with exercise. Maybe you hurt yourself while riding a bike or you did too much too soon and couldn't walk the next day. Learn from the experience, get over it and get to loving yourself enough to do what's right and healthy. That's so important, loving you. Love you enough to break unhealthy habits and/or at least add in a few healthy ones.

Another thing to do is make exercise fun. Do it with your spouse, a buddy, someone you enjoy hanging around. Make it a good memory, something to look forward to. If you don't have any friends, it's time for a change. Life is way more fun shared with other people.

I DON'T HAVE TIME!

This is a big one. **Everyone has 24 hours daily**. You can find time to do important things; you just have to set your priorities.

Maybe you don't have time to drive to the health club, work out, drive back home and prepare to go to work. Take your clothes with you and prepare for work at the club. It just takes a little planning. If that is too much, work out at home.

Maybe you need to get up a half hour earlier every day. Do it. Most folks who exercise regularly sleep harder. You'll sleep so much better; you won't even miss a half hour from your day. And folks who get their exercise in early during the day tend to stick with it. (Try to get seven to nine hours of sleep every night.)

Maybe you have to get the kids ready in the morning, take them to school and make dinner at night…exercise during your lunch time at work. Or exercise while they are at school. You can do housework with them in the house. Or, set up a time with your spouse where one can work out while the other keeps the children and vice versa. If you are a single parent, find another single parent who can trade exercise time with you. Or you can put your children on a schedule. Their nap time is your workout time. Do not let your children dictate your schedule. It really should be the other way around. The adult has the power. Own it. Claim it. Use it.

EVERYONE can find 25 minutes daily for exercise. If you ever sit and watch television, you have time to exercise. If you are into television that much, workout while the TV is on; just make sure you pay attention to your workout intensity. Just watching television can be a waste of time. And I am a TV junkie, so I get it. But we must get our priorities in order.

I'M EMBARRASSED BECAUSE OF MY SIZE

Why do we think everyone is looking at us? Most folks are too busy thinking about themselves to notice anyone else. If someone is paying so much more attention to you, he/she is probably a good partner candidate or they need to get a life.

Do this test. Ask someone you see regularly, but are not close to, "what did I wear yesterday?". Ask someone like the mail carrier, the bus driver or the server at the donut shop or an office mate. Bet they don't know... get my point?

Well, just in case you don't...

The point is not to care about what other people think. This you do for you. You can always work out at home, but the more us normal folk are seen, the more normal it will be to see us. Be a part of the solution. Be proud of who you are and let other folks know you love yourself enough to do the right thing. If you are a little shy, there are women only/men only gyms around. Just remember, for many it is easier to stick with it when you join a group. In this age of computer shopping, banking, dating and more, we could all use a little more physical interaction. Okay… The whole coronavirus thing means interacting six feet apart or on a group video call.

I DON'T WANT TO LOOK LIKE A MUSCLEHEAD

Get real. To get the kind of body you see on the people doing infomercials, you have to work out REALLY HARD. And, you have to eat a VERY healthy diet. If you're complaining about doing the minimum amount of exercise necessary to keep healthy, you won't have to worry about becoming super-muscular. I don't care what kind of genes you have.

I DON'T LIKE TO SWEAT

Sweating is a natural, healthy thing to do. It's a sign you are stimulating the metabolism enough to make a difference. If you don't sweat when you work out, you probably aren't working out hard enough. Of course, there are different degrees of sweat. Some sweat a lot, some a little. When you sweat, it should be due to exercise intensity. If it is hot outside, you don't want to risk overdoing it and suffering from a heat stroke. Don't put on a plastic suit or a bunch of clothes to make yourself sweat. When it is warm, you should wear less clothing, make sure to be hydrated and sweat as a side effect of a good workout. You want to sweat. If you are worried about body odor, shower before you work out and use an anti-perspirant or deodorant. Sweat is good; get over it.

MY HAIR! (African-American sisters use this)

Ladies, find a way. I have the kinkiest hair known to man, currently not relaxed, and I work out daily. There are braids; weaves; headbands to soak up sweat; qualified professional stylists who can help you find a way. Your body needs it. Your spirit needs it. It's really, really, really, important. Exercise helps relieve stress; it builds self-confidence. Exercise is really, really, really important and critical to good health. You can have great looking hair and a healthy body. If you have to choose, great looking hair will not affect diabetes, high blood pressure, etc.… Once again, get priorities in order.

I HAVE ASTHMA, DIABETES, ETC...

Remember how your body works. An energy exchange is going on all the time. Even when there is a malfunction, such as asthma, diabetes, hypertension... Some exercise to keep your body working as well as it can is preferable to no exercise. Of course, you should check with your doctor for your own circumstance. More on exercise for people with special needs later.

MY FAMILY IS MY PRIORITY-- I CAN'T TAKE TIME FOR MYSELF

Way too many women use this excuse. Even some men do. The funny thing is, they think it is being selfish to take time to exercise. If you don't take care of you, who will? I am not advocating one dump their family values, but it is not noble or giving or smart of you to neglect your own health and put the blame on family responsibility. Your family wants you to live longer and healthier, even dysfunctional ones.

I DON'T KNOW, I NEVER REALLY THOUGHT ABOUT IT

Well, duh! We take our health for granted so often it's pathetic. In case you haven't figured it out, good health is not granted you just for the asking. You have to do your part. Having a healthy lifestyle does not have to consume your life, but it must have a small space in your everyday and YOU have to figure out how it's going to happen. When the evening news reported the surgeon-general has determined inactivity is detrimental to your health, you shouldn't just shrug: WAKE UP! What? You don't watch the news! You have deeper problems. Grow up and take responsibility for your body and participate in life with the rest of the world. Geez.

I GET ENOUGH EXERCISE IN MY JOB

I hear this one so much, it deserves its own chapter.

CHAPTER FOUR

An Active lifestyle vs. Exercise

Some folks think, "I walk in my job, I don't need to exercise". Or "I climb poles, I dig ditches" … Whatever.

Hey, I teach fitness classes and I still workout so my body can do its job better.

When we exercise, we are moving toward a specific goal. We are trying to make our major muscles stronger. We are trying to increase the efficiency of our heart and lungs. We stretch to lubricate the joints and lower the risk of injury. We train our bodies to do our jobs better, live our lives healthier.

A simple example: Michael Jordan, one of the best baskctball players ever in my opinion. Do you think he only played basketball? I have never trained him, but I bet he strengthened his leg muscles to jump higher. He trained his upper body muscles with exercises, not just by throwing the ball. He strengthened his heart and lungs so running up and down the court would be easier. He stretched for more agility on the court. Every great athlete does more than their sport to become a GOAT.

(Greatest Of All Time)

Okay, maybe you don't aspire to play pro basketball. Maybe you play tennis. Maybe you don't do sports. Your body still needs a balanced exercise program to keep it running efficiently and lessen the risk of injury. Doing housework doesn't cut it. Gardening doesn't cut it (pun intended).

Hah! You say. I know, I know. You've read or saw on the news or heard from your girlfriend that gardening, washing the car, housecleaning and such can be a workout. If it is, you are **really** out of shape. Furthermore, it is not a balanced program designed to strengthen your muscles, improve your cardiovascular system and increase your flexibility. Just because you are burning calories doesn't mean you are exercising. Just because you are sweating doesn't mean you are exercising. If it's 100 degrees you can sit and sweat. That's not exercise.

Truth be told, it is easier to schedule in a 25-minute exercise session than it is to try and fit it in while you're cleaning the house. Sure, if you're reaching overhead to get a cobweb, you're stretching; but your ultimate goal there is to get the cobweb, not increase flexibility. By just exercising correctly, targeting the muscles, the cardiovascular system or stretching, you get the appropriate amount and intensity of exercise and then you can continue your day.

Viewing exercise as something less important to be fit in "whenever" is the problem in the first place. Cleaning your house, tending your garden… is not more important than your health. Treat it as such.

An active lifestyle is not a substitute for regular exercise. An active job isn't either. When you fill a mailbag and walk delivering the mail; that is your job--not your exercise. You still need a strong, balanced body to keep doing your job efficiently and safely.

Sure, an active lifestyle or job burns calories. Parking across the lot instead of at the door, taking the stairs instead of the elevator… all of these strategies work if you are trying to lose pounds. Adding activity to your daily life burns more calories and for weight loss you want to burn off as many calories as possible. It is not the same as doing specific exercises to strengthen your heart, lungs and muscles and to increase your flexibility. Getting fit is not about getting skinny. You too can be fit and fat... or can you?

CHAPTER FIVE

Is It Possible to be Fit and Fat?

This is a theory, or maybe a personal opinion backed by a few facts.

FACT: An overweight person who works out regularly and correctly has stronger muscles, heart and lungs than an underweight (or normal weight according to those #@*^ charts) person who does not exercise.

Keeping this in mind, I find it easy to be fit and fat and happy. By taking the focus off of looking a certain way and keeping it on fitness and health, it's easier for me to keep going. Maybe it would be easier for you, too!

There was a time when I would never walk. I just felt it wasn't a hard-enough workout for me. If I wasn't burning at least 500 calories per hour, there was no point. Now being older and wiser, if I don't feel like running, I walk instead of doing nothing. I changed my focus from trying to lose a zillion pounds to stimulating my metabolism. I am still conscientious of getting my heart rate up. Otherwise it WOULD be a waste of time as far as strengthening my heart and lungs go. (More on training zone and Target Heart Rate (THR) and why later.)

Which brings me to the fit and fat. If you do the minimum amount of exercise necessary to keep the body strong, you will technically be fit.

FACT: When a doctor assesses whether you are in good health or not, they run a battery of tests. They may check your blood pressure, your levels of blood sugar, of cholesterol and fatty acids in the blood. You can have acceptable, even ideal levels of all these things and be overweight and unfit. The doctor might mildly suggest you lose weight, but when a doctor tells me to lose weight and all my tests come back good, do I pay her any attention? No. I should, but ya know, if it ain't broke, don't fix it. I have a theory… Many young people creep into being fat and unfit this way. And by the time unhealthy numbers due to their lifestyle show up, it is even harder to fix what's broken. Maybe it's time to redefine "broken".

When I was in high school, there was this test everyone had to pass. You had to do so many sit-ups, push-ups, run a mile so fast and more. I think it was called the President's fitness test, or something like that. It was not impossible to be overweight and pass the test.

In my opinion, body size is not an indicator of how healthy you are. If your heart is strong, works efficiently and your muscles are strong enough to get you through your life without undo effort, you are fit enough.

There are different levels of fitness. An Olympic athlete's level of fitness is different from Average Joe's because it needs to be. If you are rock climbing, you need to be able to pull up your body weight. If the toughest climbing you do is up the stairs to bed, you don't have to be able to lift your body weight. People who make their living on film need to look a certain way or they won't work (another area where major improvement could be made in depicting people as they really are). People who make their living sitting behind a computer terminal don't have to look a certain way. Comparing the two is ludicrous.

So, what is fit for Average Joe? If there were a presidential test for average adults, what would it look like? Here's my suggestion.

- *Able to run/walk a mile in 16 minutes without going into cardiac arrest. Bike it in 10. (For those unable to walk but able to ride a stationary bike.)*

- *Able to do 100 crunches in 3 minutes.*

- *Able to touch your feet while sitting on the floor.*

- *Able to do 10 push-ups on your toes.*

- *Able to push your own body weight plus 100 lbs. on the leg press machine 5 times.*

- *Able to do two pull-ups.*

If you worked out just until you could accomplish all of these tasks, you may not lose any weight. You must change your diet to lose weight. But you would be fit enough. Actually, if you are a non-exerciser and do the minimum amount of exercise necessary to stay healthy and don't change your diet, you should lose some weight, (if you are truly overweight to begin with). You may even gain weight because muscle weighs more than fat. Because of all these variables, I suggest, once again, to ignore the scale. If you must have a number as a goal, get your body fat tested and use it for comparison.

Now of course, if you weigh 300 pounds it won't be easy (at 160 lbs., pulling my weight up on a bar twice is hard but I can do it), but by starting slowly and just keeping these goals in sight it can happen. If you lose a few pounds along the way, that's great! If you NEVER accomplish the above but do the minimum exercise necessary to keep everything running efficiently, that's great! It shows you love yourself enough to do what's right for your body. If other people think you are not fit, to hell with them. You know the truth. If you are obese (don't even think about the charts, you know in your heart if you are way over-fat), you should eat less and figure out why you overeat. I'll go into detail on that later.

If you are like me and feel something has to be broken before you attempt to fix it, try passing the suggested fit test for adults. You don't get any breaks because of age, race, or hair color. If you don't pass, "fix yourself" so you do.

You are or are not fit in relation to what you need to do in your life. Even if the hardest thing you do is walk from the bed to the bathroom to the refrigerator, you need to maintain a

minimum of amount of body strength. Exercise should stimulate

the cell regeneration thing enough to keep your body in good

health, (relatively speaking) for the next 60 years or so.

Although accomplishing some of the tasks in the adult fit test

isn't easy, it isn't very hard.

Let's start with the muscles…

CHAPTER SIX

Muscle Exercise

The sure way to stimulate the muscles enough to keep your body's muscle cell regeneration at peak efficiency, is to do specific muscle strengthening exercises.

The body, (back to the energy efficient thing) gets strong in relation to the stress put upon it. So, if you NEVER do any muscle exercise, your muscles get smaller and weaker. Now it takes a while for this degeneration of the body to happen, but it does happen. If you've ever broken a limb and had to rest it for a while, muscle atrophy happens fast and is easy to see. The injured limb gets smaller and weaker and you have the uninjured limb to compare it to. When it's the whole body, it's a little harder to visualize.

To illustrate this further, let's look at your household budget. If you earn $1000 a month, you wouldn't rent an apartment for $950 a month. You would get something around $350 so you could have some financial cushion, can afford to eat and maybe even go out. Your body, on the other hand, would rent the apartment for $950 a month because it likes living on the edge. Or more accurately it only wants to work just enough.

When you do exercises to strengthen your muscles, you put muscle strength in the bank, metaphorically speaking. If you only walk for exercise, you aren't developing leg muscle strength for the bank. Consequently, if you have to walk up a flight of stairs, it's a little harder. As we get older, without strengthening exercise, we get weaker. One flight of stairs feels like climbing a skyscraper.

In my years as a group exercise instructor, I have worked at a few senior citizen homes. Many of our elderly population are unable to walk stairs, have balance problems and other maladies because throughout their lives, they never did muscle strengthening or balance exercises. To keep muscles strong, you have to do muscle strengthening exercise. "Use them or lose them", as the saying goes.

Hopefully, I've convinced you of the importance of muscle exercise. If not, think about your body. It was designed to last 130 years or so. The everyday stresses of living and modern medicine, has the average life expectancy around 78 years in the United States. If you don't exercise, your muscles won't last that long. Weak muscles have folks falling down stairs, unable to keep up their housework or yard work in their later years and/or confined to a wheelchair/walker. Of course, there is no guarantee something else won't happen to lessen your quality of life. But a strong body recovers better than a weak one. It makes sense to take control over things we can control.

If you're still not convinced, read on. Once you see how easy it is, maybe you'll come around.

As stated earlier, muscles get strong in relation to the stress put upon them. When you cause a muscle to use energy, replacement energy is sent to the muscle. Thus, stimulating the energy exchange/cell regenerating thing (maybe a little oversimplified, but you get my drift).

Every movement your body makes comes from the contraction or extension of a muscle. To effectively work out the muscle, find out what it does and add resistance to it while it's doing its thing. Repeat until the muscle is fatigued, give it a day or two of rest and it will gain/maintain strength. Pretty simple.

Let's take the arm as an easy example. The bicep (the muscle at the front of the upper arm) lifts the hand to the shoulder. It needs to be strong to carry groceries. You can add resistance by grabbing a dumbbell or resistance tubing and lifting it until you can't anymore. Do it again in two days. I suggest starting with 3 – 5 pounds and working your way up to 10 or 20 pounds for women; 25 to 35 pounds for men. How do you know when to increase the weight? If you're lifting the weight easily 30 times, increase the weight. Once you get to 25 pounds for women, 45 for men, there's no need to move up. Just keep doing the exercises to maintain your strength. If you never get to 25 or 45 pounds it's okay, just keep doing it. Once it gets boring you can add variations by changing the angle or the hand position. You must change the exercise periodically to keep the muscle responding to the exercise. Something as simple as going extra heavy for one lift could be enough. Once you feel you are not getting results or you feel as though you are losing strength, it's time to hire a private trainer or take a class. (Nothing that will ruin the budget, just one session to get a new routine.) Make sure the trainer or class instructor is certified by one of the associations respected in the industry (NASM, ACSM, ACE are three) and takes your needs into consideration.

Now it may seem strange that you have to change your routine periodically to keep getting results. The reason for that is our energy efficient body. If it does the same thing, the same way constantly, it gets efficient at doing it. It doesn't have to use as much energy to accomplish the same task. The result is, you get stronger and then plateau. A little change, every two months or so will keep the body responding to exercise. It will also keep you from getting bored. In the event you do get bored, (remember the brushing of the teeth?), do it anyway.

It is also important to work out the body symmetrically. If you work your biceps you must also work your triceps. If you work the chest, also work the back. Gravity is pulling on our bodies all the time. If one muscle group resists gravity better because it is stronger, we get out of alignment. Being just a little off can contribute to back pain, knee pain and more. And yes, we tend to have one side stronger than the other…another reason why muscle exercise is so important. It is the only way to balance out natural strength imbalances.

The entire body can be kept minimally strong with this same concept of exercises. At the end of the book are exercises for the major muscles of the body. It might take you 20 minutes to do all of them, and doing them two times a week is all that's necessary to keep up minimal strength. Keep in mind we just want to maintain enough muscle strength to carry groceries, lift small children and push the car in the snow when we are 70 years old. If you want to look like Arnold Schwarzenegger did in "Pumping Iron", that's a different book. The focus here is to gain and keep the minimal muscle strength necessary to have a healthy life.

Whether or not you decide to alter your eating behavior to look like one of the models on a gym commercial, having muscle strength is important for a healthy body. Yes, it's true; muscle requires more energy to keep up than flab and consequently raises your resting output of energy. Translation: you burn more calories while sitting in front of the television. While that is a wonderful thing, we do muscle exercises to strengthen the muscles. Any other benefits are just gravy on the potatoes or icing on the cake. In this book, the aim is to exercise because your body needs it, whatever size you are.

Well, hopefully you see the importance of muscle exercise. If you don't use it, you will lose it. And you really, really don't want to lose your muscle strength.

Even if you're 100 pounds overweight, you still want to do some muscle exercise. It is true that carrying extra weight around means your muscles work harder and actually build some strength. The difference is, they never get enough rest. Eight hours a night isn't enough. Muscles without enough recovery time get weaker. If you are carrying an extra load, you want to work your muscles so they can better handle the weight.

The same holds true if you use your muscles in your day job. When you dig ditches or climb poles or lift heavy packages, you don't work your muscles evenly. Maybe you use your quadriceps (front part of the thigh) and not your hamstrings (back part of the thigh). Remember muscle strength imbalances can cause other problems relating to posture and more because of the constant pull of gravity. This can lead to back pain, knee pain, shoulder problems and more. If you have a job where repetitive motion injuries are common, seek out exercises and/or stretches to help prevent injuries. Who do you ask? A trainer or a physical therapist. Hopefully, your employer has looked into the matter and has the information on hand. Even without specific information, you should strive to do specific, goal-oriented exercises to strengthen your muscles. Evenly... All of them...Twice a week... Minimum.

Once again, I hope I've convinced you of the importance of doing muscle exercises; not to look like a muscle-bound beach bum, but to be strong enough to live your life, in its eternity, healthily. Not that being a muscle-bound beach bum is a bad thing. Living on the beach probably is a lot of fun. Ahh, moving on...

CHAPTER SEVEN

Cardio-vascular Exercise

Heart and lung exercise. We know what the heart and lungs do. Beat and breathe, respectively. Well, let's get a wee bit more detailed.

Your body needs oxygen to live. Oxygen is carried throughout the body in the bloodstream. The lungs take in air, the oxygen absorbs through special pathways to get to the heart, where it's added to the blood. (That's a very simple explanation) Then the heart pumps it through the body. Actually, the arteries and veins help move things along, but the heart is where it all starts.

The heart is a muscle. The lungs are an organ, but to keep it simple, think of them as a muscle too.

Many of the energy exchanges going on in our bodies need oxygen to happen. If you don't breathe, everything stops. If your body is not getting enough oxygen, the heart pumps faster trying to get more of the not-so-oxygenated blood through the body. The lungs then expand more often, trying to get enough oxygen, which means they are working harder. If you smoke, you are experiencing this on a regular basis. (Here is another reason to quit smoking.)

Of course, we want our heart and lungs to be strong and they get strong by working hard. But if they work hard all the time, they wear out.

Just like the muscles, the heart and lungs stay strong in relation to the stress put upon them. Your lungs supply the oxygen, which travels in the blood by your breathing two times a minute (efficient lungs) or ten times a minute (not so efficient lungs). Your resting heart pumps the blood through the body at 50 pumps per minute (a strong heart) or 100 beats per minute (not so strong). These numbers are for comparison only.

A strong heart-lung combo works efficiently. It can give a good strong pump (heart) moving easily oxygenated blood (courtesy of very efficient lungs) and consequently not have to work so hard.

When we do cardiovascular exercise, we make the system work harder (the lungs inhale/exhale more often and the heart beats faster) and then we give it a rest. That's how to make the heart and lungs stronger and more efficient. You need to do this for 20 consecutive minutes, *minimum*, at your Target Heart Rate (THR) or close to it, to get the benefits. Walking, running, cycling, dancing… any rhythmic, repetitive action using the large muscle groups will work for cardio-vascular strength. They have lots of cardio machines: steppers, treadmills, bicycles and more. You can get one for the home or go to the gym and use a different one each month. Just do it three times a week, 20 minutes minimum (add at least 3 minutes for a warm up and remember to cool down at the end for at least 2 minutes) at your Target Heart Rate.

Target Heart Rate (THR) is the level of stress to the cardiovascular system necessary to get benefits. An obese person can walk at two miles an hour and get a good cardiovascular workout, while a person at a "normal" weight might not break a sweat at that pace. Knowing your THR will help you determine if you should stick to a 2 mph walk or crank it up to 5 mph. There are two popular, easy to do ways to determine it.

The first is a percentage of your Maximum Heart Rate (MHR). Your MHR is the maximum beats per minute (bpm) your heart can stand before the danger of heart attack is too high. This number is found (and this is not absolute, it is a ball park figure) by subtracting your age from 220. If you are 30 years old your MHR is 190 bpm. Anywhere from 50 to 90 percent of 190 beats could be your target heart rate. You can determine the percentage by assessing your fitness level. If you have not worked out since a Bush was in office, you start at the 50% level and work your way up. There is no need to go above 80%, unless you're training for the Olympics or something.

The second way to determine THR is with the perceived exertion scale. You rate how hard you are working out by if it feels very easy, moderately hard, hard or very, very hard. Now, I have seen people who say they are working very hard and they ain't even broke a sweat. They aren't breathing hard and they're talking to me like they're on the phone. Don't cheat yourself. This method is best if you are taking medication to lower your blood pressure or if you are pregnant.

There is also a stress test, which is performed by your doctor or a fitness specialist at some health clubs. While you are working out on a treadmill or stationary bike, your blood pressure/heart rate is taken. The load is increased (the treadmill increases speed and/or incline or the resistance is increased on the bike) and your physical response is measured. Using this information along with your history, a much more accurate THR can be determined.

Whatever method you use to determine if you are working at your THR, know that you should be sweating, breathing a little harder, but not out of control (as in panting with mouth open) and it should actually feel good.

FEEL GOOD? AM I CRAZY?

No, I am not crazy. When you work out the cardiovascular system at the correct intensity long enough (it's different depending on the person and the activity) feel-good endorphins are released into the system. Your body needs exercise and when you exercise properly and roll with the flow, so to speak, it feels good. Your body is designed that way, so you'll keep up the exercise. Have you heard of runners high? It is not a myth, but you may be dancing or riding a bike. If you overdo it, you may hurt yourself and since you're sore afterward, you don't like the experience. Once you find the right aerobic activity at the right intensity, it will feel good. I promise you.

Back to aerobic activity… Once again, it is any rhythmic motion using the large muscle groups that elevates the heart rate. Brisk walking, jogging, running, skating, cycling, stair climbing, dancing, rope jumping and aerobic classes are some examples. Swimming can be one, but you have to be in really good shape to swim at your THR for 20 minutes straight.

Hopefully, after reading how easy and important cardiovascular exercise is to your body, you will find an activity you like and do it—three times a week, 20 minutes in a row, minimum.

What happens if you don't? Well, as stated earlier, if you don't use it, you lose it. The heart muscle, like any other muscle, only works as hard as it has to. If you are a couch potato, eventually you will only *be able* to be a couch potato.

If the hardest thing you do is walk to the store, eventually you won't be able to because the heart works to stay just strong enough.

If you are training to win a 3-mile race, you practice running 5 miles, so 3 miles is very easy to your body.

Over time, if the heart is not exercised to be strong, it becomes weak. A weak heart cannot pump efficiently, so it has to work harder. If it has to work hard all the time, it will send a signal to your brain, "hey, I can't hang, don't do so much". Consequently, the body does less; it's too tired to do any more.

Let's take another look at the aging population. Why is it some 80-year old folks can go to the gym, dance and still function and some can't. It's because of the way they have taken care of their bodies and genetics, but let's look at the things we can control. If one works to keep the heart and lungs strong, they will work more efficiently and ultimately last longer.

In an effort to see just how little is needed to be effective, studies have been done which indicate working out in short bursts throughout the day can give good results. I recommend doing 20 minutes consecutively because it is too easy to skip shorter sessions and too intrusive to exercise 2 or three times a day. I also think, (ALERT! this is MY THEORY), consecutive minutes better condition the veins and arteries. This smooth muscle tissue expands slightly during exercise and the rushing blood helps "clear the pipes". On the other hand, if short spurts of cardiovascular activity work for you—go for it.

And because we want to keep the joints moving smoothly…

CHAPTER EIGHT

Flexibility Exercises

When some folks think of flexibility, they imagine Misty Copeland lifting her leg to her head while standing tall or jumping in the air and doing splits. Let's come back to earth.

Everyone has his or her own level of flexibility. Some people can touch their toes, some can't. The point is to stretch as far as your muscles and joints will allow you to on a regular basis.

When stretching, you must warm up first. I have seen many people go to the track, stretch and then run. WRONG. Imagine your joints are like bubble gum. If you want to blow a bubble, you have to chew the gum first. Your muscles need to move around to get the juices flowing before you can stretch safely and effectively. Or let's take a rubber band. Put it in the freezer for five minutes and then try to stretch it. Got it?

Translation. Before you play tennis, jog a half-mile and then stretch your hamstrings, quadriceps, calves, shins, triceps, shoulders, back and chest. Same with basketball or any sport you are playing.

When doing cardiovascular exercise, most activities do not require you go through a full range of motion—unlike sports where a full range of motion can help a tennis player deliver a killer serve. If you're just doing cardio, you can do your entire 25 minutes (remember the warm-up) and stretch the entire body afterward.

When stretching, you figure out the two points where the muscle attaches to the bone and gently move against it. Hold the stretch for about 20 seconds. Do not bounce and it should be relaxing.

Let's look at the hamstring, which is located at the back of the thigh. To stretch it, put your heel on an elevated surface (like a curb or ballet bar, the higher the surface the more flexible you are) and lean forward at the waist. Keep the knee joint softly straight. Do not lock the knee joint.

There are stretching exercises at the end of the book. I suggest you stretch after every workout you do, muscle or cardiovascular. There are stretching classes and I think it's the safest way to learn proper stretching technique. Videos work too.

Stretching should never hurt. Relax with it. If you are "tight", it might be a little uncomfortable, but if you stay within your own limits, it should feel good. Not as good as the cardiovascular "feel good", but a relaxing, calming "feel good".

If you don't do anything else, get in some stretching exercises. I find it is a good, safe way to start an exercise routine. The muscles are stimulated, the joints are kept healthy and it is easy to do. Warm-up first and just hit every joint on the body.

How many joints are there in the body? 360. Let's just deal with the major ones.

First of all, a joint (on the body) is anywhere two bones connect. We want to stretch the ones that help us move. There are actually bone connections in the head but we don't stretch them. The shoulder, the knee, the elbow, ankle, hip… You get my drift. When we stretch the tendons and ligaments get super "lubed". Walk around the block a few times, not hard enough to get to your THR (although why not), come home and stretch.

I didn't mention bones earlier, I think I'll do it now…

CHAPTER NINE

Dem Bones, Dem Bones

I am not aware of anything like "bone exercises", but bones are a very important part of our bodies. They also have a cell-regenerating thing happening on a regular basis and need stimulation to keep them strong. Now I am getting into my theory territory.

Bones keep strong in relation to the stress put upon them and therefore need a little impact activity to maintain strength. I have a friend who had her bone density checked and was surprised to find it was low. She exercised all her life and took calcium supplements. However, I noticed in class whenever I did a jumping move, she would opt for the non-jumping version. Now, there may be some other explanation for her bones not being as dense. Eating a lot of protein (calcium is excreted when your body processes it), having children (she had four), who knows. Bottom line, a little high-impact activity in her workouts may have coaxed her bones into being stronger.

I suggest everyone who is able incorporate a little high impact activity into his or her workouts. Persons who suffer from osteoporosis or any bone problems obviously cannot do any high impact activity, but if your bones can handle it, a little impact activity should make them stronger, in theory.

I came to this conclusion by observing fish; yes, fish. Well, not really. I think they are actually mammals as I was watching whales. But you can notice the same thing in fried catfish. Fish or any creature that lives in water has exceptionally strong muscles and their bones are flexible, tough cartilage. They never have impact activity and so their "bones" aren't hard and rigid. They don't have to be. They have adapted to their environment.

Other body parts respond to stress by getting stronger, why would human bones be any different? Muscle exercise, while helping support the join, doesn't do much for bone strength. What does one do to keep the bones strong? Bone exercise! No such thing. Okay, impact activity to let the bones know they have to be strong to keep from breaking. High impact means stronger bones. Low impact means somewhat stronger bones.

No impact, means no stimulation of the bones and hence no bone strength gains.

A little impact activity can go a long way in strengthening the bones. High impact exercises like jumping rope and running are for those who aren't obese and are somewhat fit. The force of gravity when doing high impact activities is too much stress for bones that have to carry a heavy load. Low impact exercises like skating and walking are for those who can't run and jump (but are working their way up to it). Non-impact exercises like swimming and cycling do not stimulate the bones and are great for those who cannot do any jarring activity. If swimming and cycling are your favorite aerobic activities you can try running in the pool or mountain biking in rough terrain to add gentle impact. The trick is to add just enough bone jarring activity to keep the bones strong. Because I am in my theory category, an adequate amount has not been established. I think two to three minutes of jarring, three times a week should do it. Of course, not three days in a row; give the bones recovery time. The cell turn-around thing means you get a new skeleton about every

10 years. So, jump around… jump around… jump up, jump up and get down.

Now, let's get a routine going. If you have never liked exercise, start easy. If you have never exercised, start easy. Because you are *starting*, start easy. Ease exercise into your life, the risk of injury is low, it's easier to stick with, and it is easy…

CHAPTER TEN

Easing Exercise into Your Lifestyle

This is one area where many folks think it will just happen.

IF YOU DON'T PLAN IT, IT WON'T HAPPEN.

Think of everything in your life that is routine. Everyone has a morning routine. Some folks get up, drink coffee, read the paper, shower and go to work. Some get up, get in the shower and head out the door. Everyone has a plan. Others eat breakfast or they can't function, some skip it because the thought of eating that early in the morning is unthinkable (not the healthiest way to start, but I'll talk about that later). There are evening routines too. Some read before going to sleep or eat a meal before crashing, (another unhealthy habit I'll deal with later).

These routines didn't happen overnight. They developed as you developed as an individual. Your exercise routine is going to need a little help getting established. If your approach to exercise is "well...I'll work out if I have a free moment; when daylight savings time changes and my kids get into school and the wars around the world end", you aren't serious about it.

GET SERIOUS!

You need to rethink your routine. If your hours are sporadic, your plan might be: Whenever I get up, I allow 30 minutes for exercise, 25 minutes for grooming and go on with my day. If you are an evening person, your plan might be: when I get off work, I go straight to the gym for 30 minutes and then do whatever else, including hanging out with friends. If you use a calendar, *ink*, in your workouts and schedule things around them. Bodies function better when they get up, exercise, eat and retire at the same time daily. Try it for a month and you will be surprised.

I believe if people knew how important exercise is for good health and how easy it is to do the bare minimum to keep healthy, they would make it happen. Exercise is not about losing weight. Yes, if you want to lose weight, exercise can help. But if you don't need to lose weight, you still need exercise. The Surgeon General has determined inactivity to be detrimental to your health. Do you know what that means? By exercising, you can cut the risk of heart disease, diabetes and other ailments. If you are in an accident, a strong body recovers better than a weak one. If you already have hypertension, diabetes, arthritis and a host of other diseases, exercise can help…

CHAPTER ELEVEN

Exercise and Disease

In case you haven't figured it out, I am a big advocate of exercise. Physical activity can help prevent a lot of illnesses and it just makes you feel good. I am not a fanatic. I realize, and you should too, there are some circumstances where exercise can hurt and not help one's condition. If you have any special condition, the smart thing to do is check with your doctor.

When checking with your doctor, be sure to ask about exercise in all areas: cardiovascular, muscular and flexibility. Sometimes you can do one safely, but not the other. Some examples:

CARDIOVASCULAR DISEASE: A weak, damaged heart may not tolerate intense cardiovascular exercise. Veins and arteries that are weak or filled with plaque cannot carry the blood efficiently and hence cardiovascular exercise may not be prudent. If you have circulation, or heart problems, check with your doctor. Usually some rehabilitative exercise is called for, but your doctor or physical therapist can guide you. Maybe you can do dynamic flexibility exercises because they are less likely to over stress the cardiovascular system. Muscle exercise might be okay as long as you remember to breathe correctly and not go too heavy on the weights. Check with your doctor and don't be afraid to ask about different types of exercise. On the other hand, don't self-diagnose and decide you are already too fat, or because you have hypertension you are not going to exercise. The body works better when we make it strong, maybe you just have to start very easy. Check with your doctor for the facts.

SICKLE CELL ANEMIA: The extra oxygen necessary for aerobic activity is too hard for the irregular shaped blood cells to transport. Muscle exercise, which doesn't use as much oxygen is okay, again not too heavy on the weight. Flexibility exercises can also be done.

CANCER: Depending on the type, exercise can actually help. A member of one of my step classes had breast cancer and participated even though she was going through

chemotherapy. She said it made her feel better to exercise.
Of course, circumstances are different for each person, but if
you are able to exercise, try it. You might like it. I have a theory;
stimulating the metabolism with cardiovascular exercise can
make the body process whatever's going through it more
efficiently, and the feel-good endorphins released make things
easier to deal with. Whatever the case, try keeping up an
exercise routine and see how it works for you.

TYPE II DIABETES. Here is a case where all types of
exercise can help manage the disease. Exercise utilizes some
of the sugar in your blood, decreasing the need for medication.
It can also help to control weight gain, very important in Type II
Diabetes. Once again, check with your doctor to make sure you
incorporate exercise with your medication program. After a
while you may need less medication.

ARTHRITIS: Flexibility, muscular and non-weight bearing
cardiovascular exercise, like swimming and cycling may be
your best choices. If you are experiencing a flare-up, you won't
be able to exercise that day, just exercise the next day. Many

studies show keeping active helps with all types of arthritis, you just have to experiment to see what works for you.

ASTHMA: Being asthmatic, I can vouch for this first hand. You can do all three exercises. Of course, if you are experiencing an attack, you cannot. There are cases of exercise-induced asthma; I get it whenever I do cardiovascular exercises in cold weather or very polluted air. I adjust my workouts when necessary and you can too. Once again, check with your doctor.

Almost everyone can benefit from some type of exercise, regardless of your size or circumstance. Get the facts from your doctor and go for it. Speaking of size…

CHAPTER TWELVE

Pleasingly Plump, Fat or Obese

There is a bit of controversy as to whether one can be overweight and healthy. I gave you my opinion. The most important opinion is yours.

EVERYBODY COUNTS!

Even if you weigh 400 pounds (clinically obese), there is nothing wrong with adopting some healthy exercise habits. Yes, you have to take precautions and the smart thing to do is to check with your doctor for guidelines. Remember how the body works, it takes in energy (calories) regenerates its cells and pushes out waste product. If you have a lot of body, your heart and lungs are working hard all the time to nourish all that extra body. Consequently, you will reach your target heart rate walking at a slower rate than someone who is mildly overweight, and that's okay.

Go to the gym, get on that treadmill and walk your twenty minutes at 2 miles an hour. If standing that long is a problem,

67

ride the reclining bike at an easy rate for 20 minutes, three times a week. Eventually you will be able to ride harder and if you want, longer. Get in your two muscle workout sessions a week. Stretch the major muscles gently after each workout. You can do the workout at home. If you never do anything more, that's okay. Work out the body you have, to make it stronger, so it can do its job better.

Regardless of your size, exercise is essential for good health. If you are bigger, exercise is MORE important. Your body is working harder and needs to be as strong as possible, especially the heart and lungs. Yes, you have to be extra careful, but the benefits are worth it. And yes, if you are obese, you should lose weight. Yes, it is harder for you. So, what!

Is life fair?

No, it isn't. Some very obese people feel it is too hard to even try. If you are one of them, *PLEASE, PLEASE, PLEASE,* reconsider.

We all have, at some point in time, suffered from the "well it's easier for them" blues. It's easy for him "cause his daddy's rich and owns the company". It's easy for her, "she doesn't weigh 100 pounds soaking wet". Then there's my favorite "she got a cook, a trainer and all the money anyone could ever need, if I had that I'd lose weight, too".

GET OVER IT!

Everyone has his or her own road. Yes, things are easier for some people, but so what? What does that have to do with you? Once again, everyone needs to exercise. If you hate to exercise, do it anyway. Just the bare minimum, 20 minutes of cardio, three times a week; muscle strengthening exercises twice a week and stretch every time you work out.

If you aren't obese, you STILL NEED TO WORK OUT! If you are not into the "workout" frame of mind, consider the bare minimum body upkeep. View it as a mandatory part of living healthy. Even if you are living an unhealthy lifestyle, add the bare minimum of exercise so your body can withstand more damage. People who smoke still brush their teeth, right? Put exercise in your frame of mind.

If you are underweight, ditto.

I spend more time encouraging overweight people to exercise in this book and in my life, because us heavyweights need it more (the encouragement, not the exercise). I am not

a psychiatrist/psychologist, but if you are obese, you are

punishing yourself. Learning to love yourself is easier said than

done but…

CHAPTER THIRTEEN

Loving Yourself

This is said so much these days it is beginning to sound trite. Don't let it be. Loving yourself is hard when you don't fit the popular trend of what is lovable. Sure, your mother tells you you're great, but she is supposed to, right? Well, not my mother. Every time she sees me, she remarks on how fat I've gotten, (but that's another book).

Morning affirmations, reading something inspiring, just saying "I love me" everyday can help. Take it a step further by doing something for you every day; like exercise. When you schedule exercise time for yourself daily, you reinforce "I love me" behavior.

"I love me" behavior is the difference between eating a slice of cheesecake and a half of a cheesecake. Eating something you like in a moderate portion is giving yourself a treat. When you overeat, it's punishing yourself.

If you like fried chicken, French fries, ice cream, basically unhealthy, but tasty food, eat a *little* of it. No, a large order of fries is not a little bit. Get a small order and don't finish it. Have a one-dip ice cream cone. You can even treat yourself daily; just keep exercising.

When you decide "okay I'm going to do this", do it with love. Don't try to run 2 miles the first time out, that's punishment. Start with 20 minutes and walk/run it. Make sure you sweat. Have fun! Make it your time to be a kid. Forget your troubles for a half hour daily. Run, jump, play—life is short, have responsible fun.

You will find exercise really lifts your mood, if you just do it. Studies have shown mild depression can be effectively treated with exercise, especially cardiovascular exercise.

Love thyself. When you truly do, you won't do anything to hurt yourself. You do what's good for you and to you. Yes, it is easier said than done and if you have a relationship problem with food and loving yourself…

CHAPTER FOURTEEN

Eating Disorders

Now, I am not a psychiatrist or psychologist. I am a fitness instructor who comes into contact with a lot of people struggling with weight issues, on the surface.

If you carry too much adipose tissue, you eat too much/don't exercise enough. It's real simple math. Too many calories in wind up as excess butt on. There are some metabolic disorders, which can cause one to be overweight, but it doesn't apply to most overweight people. If you just like good food and have a basically healthy relationship with food, you shouldn't become obese and actually become relatively fit just by following the exercise guidelines written earlier. Keep in mind I do not consider size 12 and 16 women or 36 waist men overweight. I think that is just the average size of the average American.

THAT IS A GOOD THING!

Deal with the overeating issue when you feel like it. A little healthy behavior begets a little more, healthier behavior. Maybe you don't overeat. You just have an efficient metabolism and like good food. Exercise regularly and don't worry about it. Everyone is not supposed to be thin... even people who work out regularly.

On the other hand, there is anorexia, bulimia and obesity. Any of these behaviors is very dangerous to your health and requires some professional assistance.

If you have an unhealthy relationship with food, you know you do. I had to slap myself in the face to deal with it. I still deal with it. Talking to a therapist can help. Talking to a girlfriend can help (but not one who shares your obsession with food or lack of it). Just know this...YOU ARE NOT THE ONLY ONE.

It is scary and reassuring all at once to know you are not the only person who can eat an entire package of fig bars in one sitting, and then eat dinner. Or maybe your thing is salty stuff. Potato chips with hot sauce—a 9-ounce bag—all at once. You go to the fried chicken place and order a 5-piece dinner for yourself. Or, you take advantage of the "special" and get a whole pizza planning to eat some tomorrow, but you finish it. I've been there. You always overeat by yourself. Maybe you are depressed about something, or anxious. Maybe you hate the way you look and decide for this moment, you don't care. It's time to talk to someone and/or take some self-inventory.

Starving yourself gets a lot more attention than stuffing yourself. In my opinion, these self-destructive behaviors are symptoms of the same problem; low self-esteem. Currently over 50 percent of Americans are considered overweight. Why does one feel not worthy, or good enough, who knows? There are lots of theories, from the "suffer and you'll get to heaven" to the "doing bad things makes me feel good" schools of thought.

I AM NOT IMPLYING EVERYONE WHO IS OVERWEIGHT IS CRAZY OR MENTALLY UNBALANCED. I AM NOT IMPLYING LOSING WEIGHT WILL MAKE YOU HAPPY

I just want anyone who has an unhealthy attitude about exercise and eating to… ya know…

GET OVER IT!

And while you're thinking about whether or not you want to admit to having a problem, start exercising. If you never lose an ounce, it can help your body stay as healthy as possible. And while I'm on the subject of food…

CHAPTER FIFTEEN

To Diet or not to Diet

Anyone who has ever read a diet/exercise book has heard so many different things about food. What to eat; what not to eat; when to eat; how to eat; don't mix protein and carbohydrates; don't eat carbohydrates; you don't need to drink milk for calcium…

EXHALE!

Let's get back to the basic truth. Your body takes in energy (calories), regenerates its cells and pushes out waste product. Your diet should facilitate these functions.

There are three different types of energy (calories) we eat: Protein, fat and carbohydrates. One gram of protein or carbohydrate has 4 calories and a gram of fat has 9.4 calories. Calories do count. How you choose to mix up your caloric intake is up to you. There is a minimal number of calories necessary for the body to do its regeneration thing. A simple rule of thumb; if you weigh 150 pounds, you probably should consume 1500 calories daily. Also, if you *want* to weigh 130 pounds, you would consume 1300 calories daily (which is not a lot of food). Next, you would take into account your workouts. If you do the bare minimum add another 200 calories. For example; if you want to weigh 130 lbs., you could eat 1500 calories a day and workout for at least 25 minutes (cardio or muscle) daily.

The healthy diet supplies all the vitamins and minerals you need without too many excess calories. The United States government provides suggestions and just about any diet designed to fight diseases (like diabetes or hypertension) will work. Just keep in mind you need at least, the RDA (Recommended Daily Allowance) of vitamins and minerals, enough fiber to bind up waste product, and enough water to flush toxins out and hydrate the body.

The U. S. Department of Human Health Services provides suggestions on how to eat healthy via their websites. Once, there was a food guide pyramid. Every few years the information changes... but it really doesn't. The basics are the same. Eat more vegetables and fruits, less sugar, salt and fat and not too many calories. Remember protein and dairy foods inherently have some fat in them which is usually saturated, so go lightly. Saturated fat can lead to heart disease or aggravate an existing problem. Cakes, cookies and potato chips are not healthy choices.

A diabetic diet goes lighter on the simple carbohydrates, mostly avoiding sugar and choosing high fiber foods.

A person with hypertension is advised to go low saturated fat and low sodium.

Some books say to lose weight, don't mix bread and meat; don't eat fruit after noon, eat all the meat you want; don't consume any starchy carbohydrates and don't eat after 7 p.m.

WHATEVER!

You know how to eat right: plenty of fruits and vegetables, a little meat (or protein) and very little fats and sweets. If you want to "follow" a plan, I recommend you get 25 grams of fiber a day. Fiber is the indigestible part of food eaten. There are two types; soluble (dissolve in body) and insoluble (does not dissolve in body). Split your daily intake of 25 grams between insoluble (raisin bran, whole grain bread) and soluble (oatmeal, beans,) fiber. Next, I recommend you drink at least 64 ounces of water every day. Your body is two-thirds water and uses water in its energy exchange functions. Most people walk around dehydrated and consequently feel fatigued. I also recommend you eat at least two servings of fruit and three of vegetables every day. One of the vegetables should be green and leafy, like spinach. Keep in mind a serving is only about 4 ounces; not big at all. Actually, get a food scale and weigh leafy greens once so you know what a serving looks like. Last but not least, 1000 mg. (men) to 1200 mg. (women) of calcium is needed daily.

Now I just didn't make this up off the top of my head. A long time ago, scientists figured out that the body and brain run on glucose. They also discovered it is easiest for the body to turn carbohydrates into glucose. It made sense to base the diet on carbohydrates. It was also determined a certain mix of proteins, vitamins and minerals was needed daily to help the body do its job. The body can't manufacture these items, thus, the recommendation for protein and fruits and vegetables. Then they figured out fiber was important in getting waste out of the body, as is water for keeping it hydrated. As new discoveries are made connecting nutrition and good health, the daily food requirements get tweaked every few years. There are constants and they are not subject to fads. They are: water, fiber, vitamins and minerals from fruits and vegetables and calcium. You also need a minimum amount of protein and fat. There are different ways to get all of these things, some healthier than others.

Over the years, studies have indicated most folks' diets lack nutritionally in these four areas; fiber, water, calcium and fruits/vegetables. These four items are so critical to good health, if you are lacking in just one the consequences are dire. Fiber helps bind up waste product so we can eliminate it from the body. Water is essential to keep everything flowing internally. Fruits and vegetables supply vitamins, minerals, and phytochemicals the body needs to neutralize free radicals. Calcium is needed for bones and the circulatory system.

If your diet is like the average American you should concern yourself with these four things, the rest can take care of itself. Of course, you should eat a little protein and fat daily, most folks eat too much protein and fat. If that is you, cut back or just make sure you get the minimum amount of the other stuff. Getting enough fiber is difficult unless you pay attention to the type of breads and cereals you eat. High fiber breads are made with the whole grain; check labels to see if your favorite bread complies. If it doesn't, change your favorite brand of bread. The same goes for cereal; choose one that is high in fiber, like raisin bran. By checking labels, you can tell if it's high-fiber or not. (I mix bran cereal with my favorite no fiber one, so I can have what I like with what I need.) Fiber also is found in fruits and vegetables. By having a high-fiber cereal, two fruits and three vegetable servings daily you should hit the 25-gram mark. (Especially if you eat a bowl of cereal like I do, twice the recommended serving size.) Calcium needs can be met by consuming three servings of calcium rich foods, like milk, yogurt and cheese and by having a green leafy veggie daily. If you are not going to eat properly it won't hurt you to take supplements for calcium as well as a multi-vitamin with minerals. And please, not mega amounts of vitamins and minerals. The minimum daily requirement will do. Most studies on vitamin mineral supplements don't show a real benefit from them unless you have a true deficiency, but if you *want* to take them go ahead. The most important thing is the fiber, water, fruits and veggies and calcium.

If you want to lose weight, eat half of what you normally do. I find it is the easiest way to cut calories and still enjoy what you like. Try to eat at the same time daily. The body loves structure and routine.

If you want to eat perfectly healthy, have two servings of salmon or tuna weekly (for Omega 3's, a special kind of "good" fat), eat only lean cuts of meat and throw away the skin of chicken (to cut "bad" fat and cholesterol). You can also cut your coffee consumption (if you drink it) to 8 oz or less a day or even better, drink green tea instead. Have a green salad daily for one of your vegetable servings. Only eat low fat choices of milk and cheese (if you eat milk and cheese). Only use unsaturated oils. Only eat one whole egg daily and it counts as a protein serving. Never eat sweets, drink soda or have fried foods. And watch your portions. If eating like this seems out of the question, I'm with you. Make changes where you can. Just be sure to get 64 oz of water, 25 grams fiber, 1000 mg. calcium, 2 servings of fruit and 3 servings of vegetables every day. Also, eat moderate sized meals at least twice a day.

Oh yeah, skipping breakfast. No one says you have to have a bacon, egg, pancake, juice and fresh fruit throw down every morning. If you are not a "breakfast person", just eat a little bit. A little bit is 100 to 200 calories; a piece of fruit, a cup of juice with a slice of whole wheat toast or one serving (the size recommended on the box) of high fiber cereal. Remember the metabolism thing? Your body takes in calories, regenerates its cells and pushes out waste product, even when you are asleep. When you wake, after 8 hours of no energy input, your body is running on low. Once you start moving, stimulating the energy output, you need to get a little energy in. Eating at regular intervals is important for keeping blood sugar levels balanced and helping the body run smoothly.

An example, once upon a time, if you let your car run completely out of gas, you had to put a little gas in the carburetor as well as the tank to get the car to start. Having breakfast is like putting gas in the carburetor.

Personally, I find my body runs better with a light breakfast. Very light. Sometimes I have a packet of instant oatmeal; sometimes just orange juice with pulp. I exercise in the mornings, so a stomach that's digesting food is plain uncomfortable. After my workout, I EAT. Lunch is my biggest meal. Sometimes I snack, most of the time I don't. Sometimes I have a "Sunday Sin day"; the kind of day where I stay in my pajamas, eat what I want and watch movies. I don't deprive myself and I don't stuff myself. Well, sometimes I still overstuff, when I am depressed, nervous, mad, stressing and I forgive myself afterward. The point is; I found what works for me.

Being a person who has tried silly diets, I find changing what you like to eat an incredible challenge. I have also found that you can lose weight eating what you like. No matter what you read, excess weight is excess calories. One could lose weight drinking one milkshake and a candy bar daily. All you have to do is keep the calorie count low. Of course, your body wouldn't be getting what it needs to function, but you'd lose weight and eventually, your good health.

Seriously, everyone knows they are not supposed to exist on junk food. Momma made you eat your vegetables when you were little so you could grow up big and strong. She was right then, and she's right now (although now you want to maintain, not grow). Your grandma told you to eat your oatmeal so you could have roughage to keep you regular. She was right then, and she's right now. You need fiber to bind up the waste product from your working metabolism. You need water to help flush out the waste and just keep the body hydrated.

Be wary of any diet advising you to cut out a complete food group. Bread, cereal, rice and pastas (carbohydrates many consider "bad") are not inherently high calorie foods. It's what we put on them, the type and amount we eat which makes us fat. If you eat just a serving, it won't make you fat. If you make them whole grain, it will be much easier to get 25 grams of fiber daily. Whole grain products also tend to fill you faster so you don't eat so much.

I find by just concentrating on getting 25 grams of fiber, 64 ounces of water and 2 fruit and 3 vegetable servings daily, the rest of my diet takes care of itself.

Find what works for you. If you can live on eating protein with your vegetables and not eating bread or rice ever, more power to you. Just make sure you are getting 25 grams of fiber, 64 ounces of water and 2 fruit/3 vegetables a day.

If you have diabetes, hypertension, colon cancer, eat how your doctor or dietician tells you to. I bet you'll be getting fiber, water and at least vegetables.

If you are a "carbohydrate addict" and want to eat only foods with a low glycemic index and it doesn't make you crazy, roll with it. If you must have your carbohydrates, don't eat so many of them and go high-fiber when possible.

I wrote earlier about just eating half of what you normally eat. This is the easiest way to cut calories from your diet without cutting the foods you love. Remember, if you want to lose weight, calories do count. Your body is simple and complicated simultaneously. Very simply, it is easy for your body to take fat calories and put them right on your thigh (store them as fat). It is a little more complicated for your body to take carbohydrates or proteins and turn them into fat for your thighs, but it can happen. Excess is excess. Some excesses are harder on your body than others. Excess protein is not the best thing for the kidneys. Excess refined carbohydrates are not the best thing for the liver and your insulin-making pancreas. Excess alcohol is also very bad for the liver.

Bottom line, moderation is the key. Make sure you give your body the vitamins and minerals it needs (by eating fruits and vegetables), intake enough fiber to bind up the waste and drink enough water to keep everything flowing. Then you must exercise to stimulate the cellular turnaround thing. And don't do anything in excess; only do what's good…

CHAPTER SIXTEEN

What Does a Body Good?

The body takes in energy, a bunch of different energy exchanges go on and waste product is excreted. I know, you've read that somewhere before.

To keep everything running smoothly, your body needs certain vitamins and minerals, and proteins and fatty acids. An example:

You are at the beach and you decide to make a sand castle. To do this you need sand, water, a shovel, a bucket to carry the water and some imagination.

For your body to regenerate its muscle cells, it needs certain enzymes and amino acids.

The water mixes with sand to change the consistency and make it sturdy building material. If the ratio of sand to water is not ideal, you castle will look like a shack. You won't want to post it on your social media feed.

If you don't eat the right amount of protein (which isn't a lot) or don't have the proper vitamins, minerals and carbohydrates to activate and aid the process, the muscles won't be very hardy.

The simple and complicated truth about the body is if you feed it junk, it will do its thing (which is take in energy and regenerate its cells) using junk. The result is a "junk" body.

A tragic, but easy to see example of this is the liver. If you consume too much alcohol on a regular basis, the regeneration of the liver cells is affected, changing the cellular structure into what is called a fatty liver. Once this happens, the liver cannot function properly.

To keep from getting a junk body, there is the recommended daily allowance (RDA) of vitamins and minerals. This is the minimum amount necessary to ward off having a "junk" body and contracting diseases, like rickets. If you want to have a "super" body, you may need more than the RDA. There are toxic levels of vitamin and minerals, so don't get too much of a good thing. The balance of vitamins and minerals is important too. The following chart lists a few of the essential vitamins and minerals needed regularly. Some are water soluble, which means you should try to eat them on a daily basis, because the body will run short sooner. Fat-soluble vitamins tend to hang around longer and should be consumed a few times a week.

VITAMIN OR MINERAL	AMOUNT MEN	AMOUNT WOMEN	TOXIC LEVELS
Vitamin A*	900 mcg.	700 mcg.	3,000 mcg.
Vitamin C*	60 mg.	60 mg.	2,000 mg.
Vitamin B1* (Thiamin)	1.2 mg.	1.1 mg.	Not established
Vitamin B2* (riboflavin)	1.3 – 1.7 mg.	1.1 – 1.3 mg.	Not established
Vitamin B3* (Niacin)	16 mg.	14 mg.	35 mg.
Vitamin B6 (pyridoxine)	1.3 mg.	1.3 mg.	100 mg.
Vitamin B12*	2.4 mg.	2.4 mg.	Not established
Vitamin D	15 mcg	15 mcg	100 mcg
Vitamin E	15 mg.	15 mg	1,100 mg.
Folate*	400 mcg.	400 mcg	1000 mcg.
Calcium*	1000 mg.	1200 mg.	2000 mg.
Iron*	8 mg.	18 mg.*	45 mg.
Potassium*	3,400 mg.	2,600 mg.	*varies
Magnesium	400 mg.	310 mg.	500 mg.
Selenium	55 mcg.	55 mcg.	400 mcg.
Zinc*	11 mg.	8 mg.	40 mg.

This information was culminated from the National Institute of Health website.
Recommended amounts vary according to age and circumstance, like pregnancy or disease.

If you eat a relatively healthy diet you should get these amounts without any problem. If you do decide to supplement, take a multi-vitamin/mineral with a balanced meal (one with some carbohydrates, proteins and a little fat). Vitamins and minerals need to ride into the body on the different types of calories. Mega dosing any vitamin/mineral is not smart. Vitamins and minerals work in the body synergistically and ingesting imbalances can cause problems.

If a registered dietician is available to you, make use of him or her. We go and get our hair done, or will seek a professional to do our nails but we won't make use of professional dieticians and nutritionists. There are people who do nothing but look at your food history and/or take your blood, analyze it and tell you what you need to be eating for better health. Just like any field you have to beware of quacks but good ones are out there (registered dieticians and nutritionists). One who is working out of a hospital or clinic is your best bet. Use them! If they are also selling the vitamin/mineral supplement: Be wary. A conflict of interest may have them selling you more than you need. You may think, "what the heck, I'll just pee out the extra". Your filtering organs do not need the extra work and I am sure when you think about it, there are other places to spend the extra money. Like in the fruit and veggie section of your favorite store.

Any high-quality multi-vitamin (not necessarily expensive) supplement will supply the government's Recommended Daily Amount of vitamins/minerals and more. Supplementing your diet won't hurt as long as you do not get toxic amounts of any vitamin or mineral and you take them with a meal. Your body cannot tell the difference between a "natural" and a "synthetic" vitamin, so why spend the money? If it carries the USP symbol, it should supply what the label says it contains. USP stands for U.S. Pharmacopeial Convention which is an organization who evaluates supplements. They check for things like: Does the contents match the label? Is it made in a clean and safe environment? They also investigate how things are sourced and more. If you just want to have designer vitamins, more power to you.

What has not been established is the RDA for herbs. Which brings me to the next chapter…

CHAPTER SEVENTEEN

What Doesn't a Body Good?

Nowadays, herbal supplements are the "in" thing. Who knew smoking blunts could cure headaches, asthma, cancer, arthritis… **JUST KIDDING!** There are herbal remedies which promise to give you more energy, help you remember where you put your keys, relax you, etc.

There is not an established RDA for herbs that I'm aware of. Personally, if I need more energy, I check my diet to make sure I'm covering all the vitamins, minerals and water I need. Then I make sure I get enough sleep. If those things are okay, I go to the doctor, to see if anything else is wrong. If I seem to forget where I put my keys, I make it a point to put them in the same place every time. If I need to relax, I take a vacation, read a book, meditate…

The point is, unless there is something wrong, taking herbs is like taking unnecessary medicine. Yeah, it's natural, but that doesn't mean it's harmless. Poison ivy is natural, too. If you think you need herbs for some malady, get educated and not from the same company who sells the stuff. More and more, doctors are embracing herbal remedies and there are homeopathic doctors. See if your community hospital or regular medical doctor can recommend a few. Once you find a homeopathic doctor be sure to inform him/her of any medications you are taking so they can be aware of any drug interactions.

Always keep in mind how your body works. Whenever you ingest anything, it interacts with the cellular regeneration thing going on in your body. Everything has an effect, and it can be good or bad or neutral. Extra work for your system needs to be measured against the benefit. Your liver and kidneys have to work extra to flush excess vitamins, medications and these organs do not need extra work.

If you suffer from anything, get advice to find out why. If you are tired, find out why. Maybe you are trying to do too much. Maybe you are dehydrated and need to drink more water. Many people are chronically dehydrated and don't know it. Once you find the cause of your problem, fix it, if possible. Trying to medicate yourself, with herbs or other things, without professional help reviewing all parameters is not the healthiest or smartest thing to do and can be harmful.

Herbs are strong medicines that should be used responsibly and can be very good for the body.

Once you realize what you need and what you don't need, how do you know what each food has in it?

CHAPTER EIGHTEEN

Reading Labels

There are all kinds of legitimate, useful information available regarding eating right. It isn't as clearly marked as it could be, but with a little guidance, making healthy food choices can be easy.

What is eating healthy? You know the answer. In case you forgot, it's eating foods that supply your body with the vitamins, minerals and calories necessary to keep it healthy. My personal way to remember is to eat 25 grams of fiber, 64 ounces of water, 1000 mg of calcium and two fruit, three vegetable servings daily. The government has guidelines to help you. Some folks recommend getting 20 – 30 percent of calories from fat, 50 – 60 percent from carbohydrates and 20 – 30 percent from proteins. Some say 30 – 40 protein, 30 – 40 carbohydrate and 30 fat. How do you know what you're getting once you decide what you want to eat?

Let's start with labeling on food. Most foods list the number of calories (energy) a serving has, the size of a serving and what type of energy (fat, carbohydrate or protein) it is. It also lists the vitamins and minerals the item has. If it isn't listed, (for example, there is not a label on an apple), the information should be somewhere in the store for you.

The label lists nutrition information as a percentage of the Daily Value or the actual amount of the item. Depending on the size of the item, the label can be horizontal and may not list everything. The important information you need to make a healthy choice is there: Calories, grams of fat, carbohydrates and protein and sodium content and amount of cholesterol. Here is an example of a label.

Nutrition Facts

About 9 servings per container

Serving size 1/4 cup (40g)

Amount per serving

Calories 120

	% Daily Value*
Total Fat 0g	**0%**
Saturated Fat 0g	**0%**
Trans Fat 0g	
Cholesterol 0mg	**0%**
Sodium 10mg	**0%**
Total Carbohydrate 31g	**11%**
Dietary Fiber 2g	**6%**
Total Sugars 26g	
Includes 0g Added Sugars	**0%**
Protein 1g	

Vitamin D 0mcg 0% • Calcium 20mg 2%

Iron 0.7mg 4% • Potas. 300mg 6%

* The % Daily Value (DV) tells you how much a nutrient in a serving of food contributes to a daily diet. 2,000 calories a day is used for general nutrition advice.

I think it would be simpler if food labels just stated how much in grams of an element it had. For example, a milk carton label should read "an 8-ounce serving of milk provides 300 mg of calcium". Instead of the percentage of the daily value, which says 30 percent. Well, if your daily value is 1200 mg of calcium, 300 mg is only 25 percent. And the calcium amount doesn't change because you need more. Then again, I am math challenged. If it works for you, cool.

Another thing to be aware of is the amount of a particular item in a food. Let's look at juices. First ingredient on most is water. If the second is high fructose corn syrup, it's got a lot of simple sugar, compared to one whose second ingredient is orange juice from concentrate. The rule is; the ingredient there is most of comes first and so on. So, if you buy a pasta dish with broccoli and dehydrated broccoli is the last item in the ingredients list, it does not count as a serving of vegetables.

Speaking of serving size. A serving is 1 to 4 ounces depending on the food. With bread and cheese, it's one to two (1-2) ounces. Not very much. Pay attention to serving size on labels and then to how much you actually eat. You might be surprised. I find I eat at least two servings of cold cereal according to the serving size on the label. And when I eat rice or pasta, even if it is whole grain, I eat more than the 2-ounce serving recommended on the label. Measure a "serving" once to get a visual idea of how much it looks like.

CHAPTER NINTEEN

EATING FIT PHAT HAPPY STYLE

I am nobody's chef. I started cooking because the food on the street is full of stuff I don't want to eat. Ingredients like salt, fat, sugar… these things taste great, but wreak havoc on the body. I found it is possible to lower the amount of salt fat and sugar and still have good food. All it takes is a little imagination, lots of spice and time. The one thing no one seems to be able to spare.

Time can be spent in many ways and cooking needs to be up there with exercise when it comes to your priorities. The cool thing is, just like the bare minimum of exercise, you can do the bare minimum of cooking. I almost always cook everything in a skillet. A lean protein like ground turkey, a bag of mixed veggies, a tablespoon or two of olive oil and a squeeze of lemon or lime and spices… done. If you switch up the spices, it stays interesting enough for everyday eating. I can get a meal on the table in 20 minutes. I shop a few times a week and do meal prep so I can have healthy food whenever I want it.

If you don't want to cook, there are ways to get around the extra salt, fat, sugar and calories found in restaurants and fast-food joints. Always ask for sauces on the side and order from the "heathy" menu, if one is available. Only eat half of whatever you order, that cuts the sugar, salt, fat and calories 50 percent and doubles your spending budget. Make some ground rules and stick to them. Maybe you only have fries once a week. Have a day of veggies only. Intermittent fasting is a way to eat less and be healthy. And then you can add in your "treats".

Some folks like to have a cheat day, but that implies it is wrong or bad to eat what you want.

Bump that.

You are a grown up and you can eat whatever you want. The hope is you WANT to be healthy, so you eat healthy. One slice of cake, one doughnut, one glass of wine or a martini… Moderation is the way to enjoy all the culinary treats this world has to offer and enjoy them you should. You just can't do them all in the same day. Budget your meals, just like you budget your money. Get the basic needs (2 fruit/3 vegetables, 25 grams of fiber, calcium and water, in case you've forgotten) and then eat what you want. If you eat the necessary stuff first,

you, theoretically, won't have room for the unhealthy stuff.

Alright already...let's do it...

CHAPTER TWENTY

Living Fat and Happy

I hope you take the information in this book and put it into action. Adding exercise to one's life is an easy way to help lessen the risk of contracting some diseases, have fun and increase self-esteem. Oh yeah, did I talk about that?

Aside from the natural high cardiovascular exercise can give, a sense of accomplishment is yours daily when you stick to an exercise program. Especially on days when you just don't feel like it.

Completing your exercising routine is totally within your control and the sense of "I came and I conquered" is so satisfying. Let's face it. Not too many areas in life offer that. If you are in sales, sometimes you make the sale, sometimes you don't. If you're an artist, sometimes your work is a hit; sometimes you are the only one who "gets it". With an exercise routine, you can always go out and do your 25 minutes of lifting, aerobics and/or stretching.

Establishing a daily exercise routine reinforces healthy behavior. If you do something good for yourself daily, you are less likely to do something bad. If you have an addiction issue, regular exercise is a tool to have in your "keep focused on a healthy lifestyle kit". It's a great way to say "I love me" daily.

Remember: Do not do the exact same thing daily. In this instance, variety is the spice of life. I find it easy to alternate cardio and muscle workouts. Once you get into it, you might find you want to take it pass the bare minimum necessary to be healthy. Maybe push your cardio workout to 30 minutes. Go for it, gradually. Keep in mind, even if you get bored, it's like brushing your teeth. The bare minimum is necessary and it doesn't have to take more than 25 minutes.

One thing for sure, whether you lose weight or not, physical activity is essential for optimal health. Muscular, cardiovascular and flexibility exercise is the best way to stimulate the body to regenerate strong and healthy.

When you plan a program and stick to it, your body and your spirit will thank you. And remember, you aren't going to live forever anyway. So, if you hear or read or wonder if you should stress about trying to lose weight because it is unhealthy;

don't worry about it. Stressing out over stuff is unhealthy and

will kill you too! Just keep exercising and glow with the fact that

you are living fat and happy.

WHAT'S GONNA HAPPEN GONNA HAPPEN ANYWAY?
NO!

You may think it's too late. Maybe you are already diabetic,

(type 2--not 1). Maybe you already have hypertension (high

blood pressure) or prehypertension

(almost high blood pressure). Maybe your arteries are already

stuffed with plaque and you don't feel like you can't change

anything. Take a moment and breathe. One really cool thing

about the body is it is always trying to heal itself. There are

instances when the body "rights" itself with just a little diet and

exercise change. A 5% decrease in weight can get your blood

pressure back to normal or lower the amount of medicine you

need to control it. Eating oats daily for 6 weeks can lower your

cholesterol enough so you don't have to take medicine or take

a lower dose. Some people can control their diabetes with diet

and exercise.

NEVER STOP TRYING!

We all have thought "to hell with it" at one point in time. When you want to give in, remember to be grateful for the ability to be. For the opportunity to make a choice, and for life. Everyone has a reason to live, otherwise you wouldn't be here. It is your job to figure out what it is. And if you need a plan or blueprint...

CHAPTER TWENTY-ONE

FOLLOW THIS

I prefer you come up with your own plan because you are more likely to follow it. You know what you like to eat, what you like to do, your strengths and your weaknesses. But if you want to do something to improve your fitness and your health that definitely works; here it is…

Walk 30 minutes at a brisk pace daily before noon.

Walk 20 minutes at a brisk pace daily after 5 pm

Every Monday, Wednesday and Friday, at the same time of day, do 20 push-ups, 30 squats, 10 pull-ups, 30 crunches and 20 back extensions.

Every day after your evening walk, touch your toes, stretch your quadriceps, upper back, sides and neck.

Simple. And if you need a little more instruction, keep reading.

CHAPTER TWENTY-TWO

Exercises for the Body

It's best to start with a whole-body warm-up. Just move around for three (at least) to ten (ideal) minutes. Every movement your body makes is the contraction or extension of a muscle. So, if you march in place while raising and lowering your arms, that'll do it. Might look a little silly, but who cares. Your exercise time is yours to become a kid again. Remember when we were kids how we would have fun, oblivious to what we were wearing or what we look like? If you've forgotten, go to a park and observe. You might see that weird kid who has already been tainted… the one who does care what others think. Look past that one. Most kids are carefree

Okay, now that you're warmed up, what to do? There are LOTS of ways to work out the body. Some exercises use a few muscles at a time; some exercises work them individually. If you are crunched for time, obviously you'll want to work a few muscles at a time. As a matter of fact, there are 5 exercises that work the major muscles--just enough. They are: *squats, push-ups, pull-ups, abdominal crunches and back extensions.* Whether you do exercise that works one muscle at a time or two or three, make sure you exhale when you exert energy. Do not hold your breath. Do enough repetitions to feel fatigue so you get the benefits of the exercise. Fatigue is the point where you just can't do another lift, squat or curl—whatever the exercise calls for. The muscle should feel the "burn" <u>after</u> you've done several repetitions. If it hurts right away, stop and get professional help so you don't injure yourself.

Speaking of injuring yourself. Please remember to stretch after working out. Even if you just hit the major joints, take five to 10 minutes EVERY DAY to stretch.

Once these exercises get easy or you have to do three times the recommended amount to feel fatigued, hire a trainer to design a more difficult program or take a class. Remember, the body adapts to whatever you do regularly and you need to challenge all those cells to keep them positively responding.

THE SQUAT

Stand with knees over ankles, hips over knees… in other words, stand up straight. Do not lock knees.

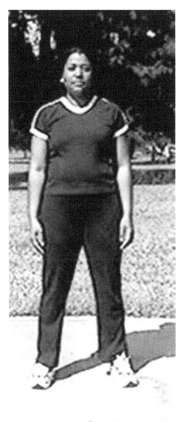 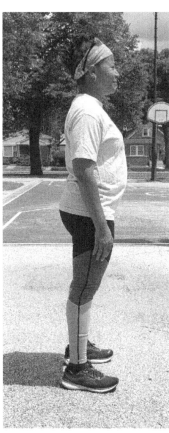

THE SQUAT 2

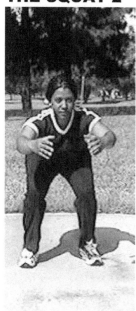 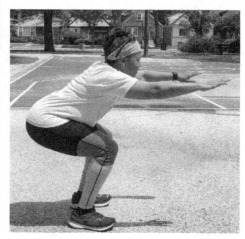

Bend your knees and lower your butt as though you were sitting in a chair. Keep your knees behind your toes and extend your arms forward for balance. Do not let knees splay in or out.

PUSH-UPS

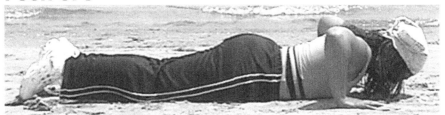

Lay on the floor face down with hands under your elbows and just below your shoulders. Hold abdominal muscles tight and keep the body straight as you push up.

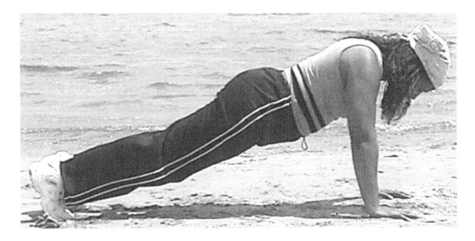

MODIFIED PUSH-UP

If a full body push-up is too difficult, you can do them on your knees or against a wall.

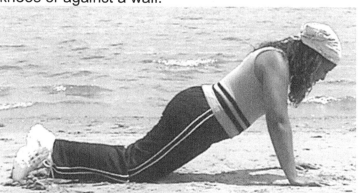

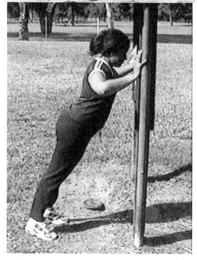

PULL-UPS

This move works the opposite muscles of the push-up. They are hard for most people. Assist your back muscles with your legs on a low bar.

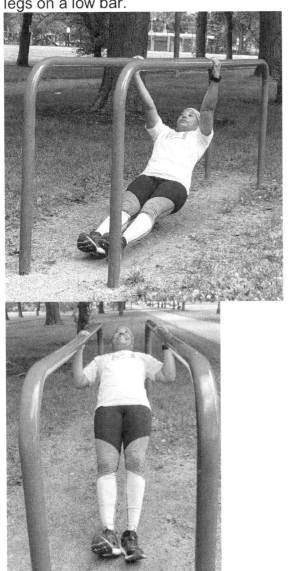

CRUNCHES

The abdominal muscles need to be strong because they hold you up. Lay on your back with knees bent and feet flat on floor. Support head with your hands. Do not pull on your head and neck. Contract abdominal muscles by squeezing navel to back. Exhale as you lift chest up and try to get upper shoulders off the ground. Return to start.

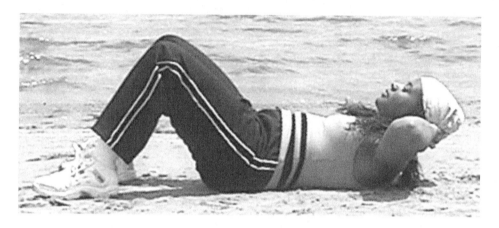

OBLIQUE CRUNCHES

Start on your back with knees bent and curl up, this time leading right shoulder to left knee and then reverse it.

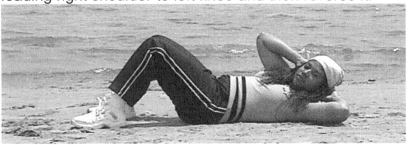

BACK EXTENSIONS

Lie face down with arms overhead. Lift the upper and lower body using your lower back muscles.

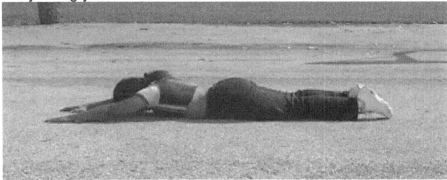

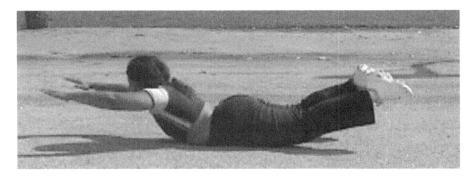

CALF AND SHIN STRETCHES

The lower leg muscles should be stretched regularly to aid in circulation and let's face it... We use our legs a lot (or at least we should). Stand with left leg behind you. Bend right knee, keeping left leg straight and heel on the floor. Hold for 20 to 30 seconds. Then put the toe on the floor, lean forward and feel the shin stretch. Switch legs.

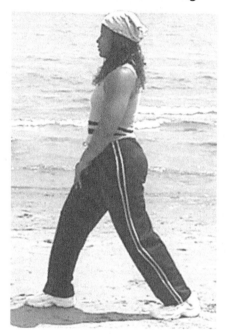 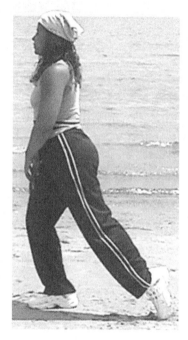

QUADRICEPS STRETCH

Stand on right leg with the left hand holding the left leg close to the buttocks. Hold 20 to 30 seconds and work your "balance muscles" by not falling over.

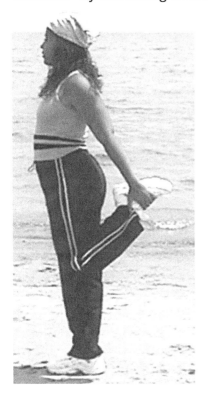

HAMSTRING STRETCH

Place right heel on a higher surface. The higher it is, the deeper the stretch, so do what you can. Lean forward at the waist with the knee straight as possible.

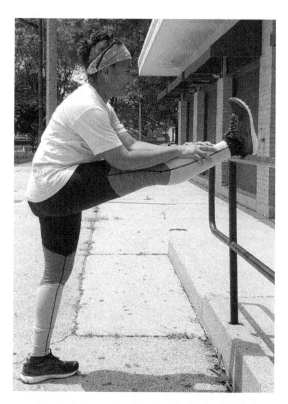

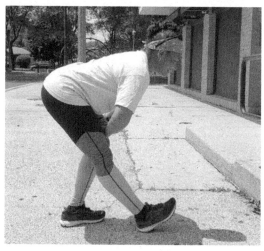

CHEST AND UPPER BACK STRETCHES

Place right hand behind and above the shoulder as shown. Turn away and feel the stretch in the chest muscles. Then turn around, hold both arms around pole or with each other and round out back.

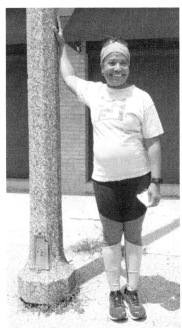
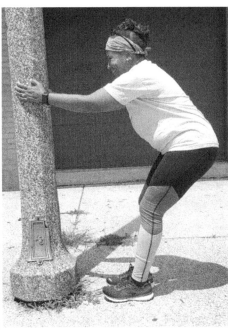

TRICEPS STRETCH

Raise right arm overhead and use left hand to press elbow back and slightly left.

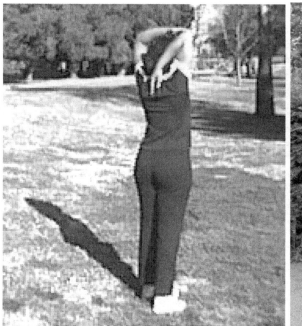
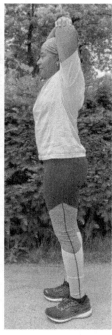

BICEPS/FOREARM/WRIST STRETCHES

Extend right forward without bending elbow. Grab fingers and thumb with palm facing up, fingertips down. Hold 20 seconds, then flip palm down and gently press palm to body. Then flip palm out with fingertips up and hold.

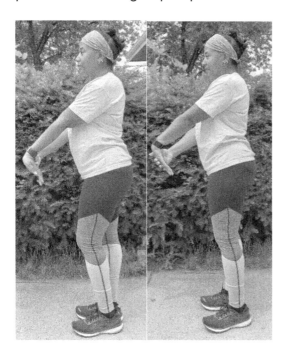

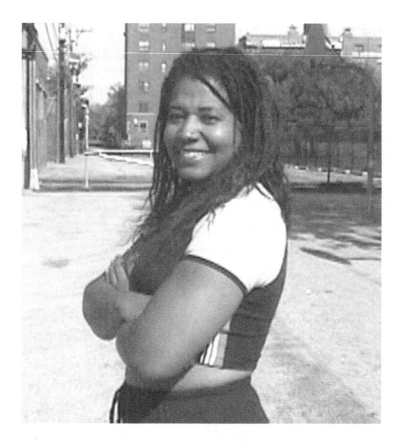

USEFUL INFORMATION

You may wonder, where did I get all this information from. Well, as part of my certification, I have to keep learning and I read A LOT. Some of my favorite are:

The Mayo Clinic Newsletter

The New England Journal of Medicine

Consumer Reports

Nutrition Action

National Institute of Health

These publications review research and print articles. I read their articles and most times look at the research papers and form my own opinion. You can check that out at my website www.fitfathappy.com. I hope you read and learn and form your own opinion and decide to take action and live your healthiest life. It is not rocket science—YOU GOT THIS!

Made in the USA
Las Vegas, NV
22 November 2020

11296941R00069